10-DAY RAPID WEIGHT LOSS DIET COOKBOOK

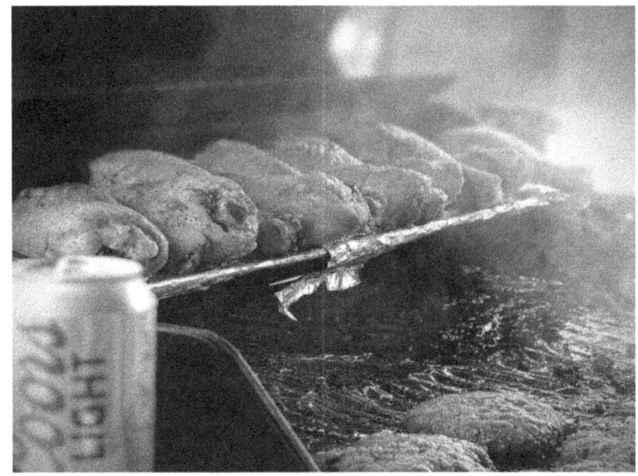

A SIMPLE 10-DAY DIET PLAN TO REDUCE BELLY FAT AND GENERATE QUICK, LONG-LASTING HEALTH RESULT!

LEAH WASHINGTON

TABLE OF CONTENTS

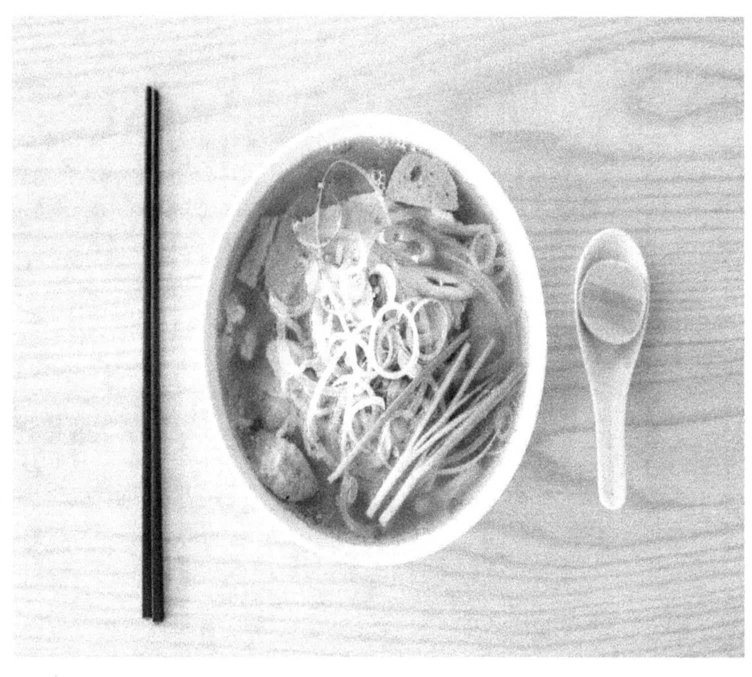

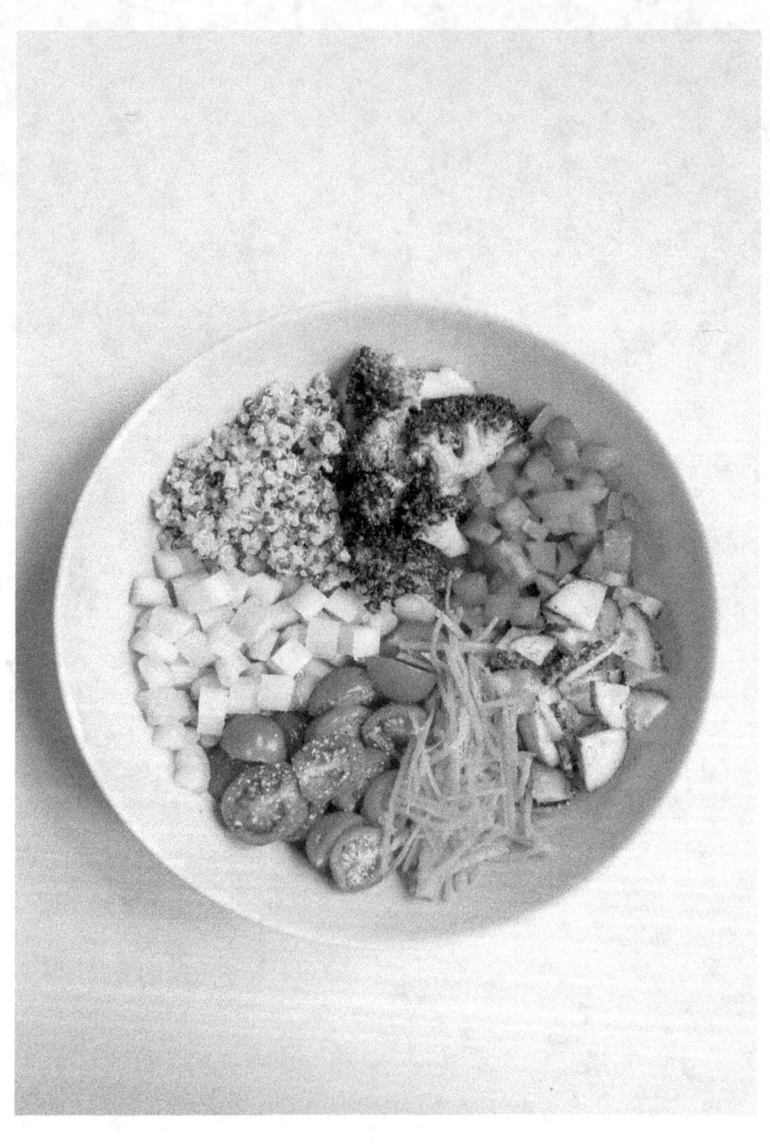

INTRODUCTION

Welcome to "Trim in Ten," where we'll set out on a transformational journey using a thoughtfully chosen 10-day food plan to lose weight quickly. With the help of this cookbook, you may effectively and sustainably reach your fitness objectives by combining delicious meals with the science of nutrition for Rapid Weight Loss.

Introducing Jane, a driven professional on a tight schedule who is determined to regain her energy. Disappointed with fad diets and unattainable food plans, she stumbles across a gastronomic journey that alters the course of events. Our cookbook serves as her guide, taking her through ten days of delectable,
meals rich in nutrients and intended to help lose weight quickly.

Every day begins with a thoughtfully planned menu that is a symphony of flavors and colors that fill

Jane up and give her energy. The meals, which range from colorful salads full of antioxidants to satisfying dinners loaded with protein, are about enjoying the process rather than just losing weight.

As Jane turns the pages, she discovers that the clever blending of materials, rather than starvation, holds the key to success. The cookbook turns into a dependable friend, transforming her kitchen into a well-being haven. Anyone looking to improve their lifestyle will feel empowered by the 10-day Rapid Weight Loss Cookbook, which offers doable meals, shopping lists, and helpful advice.

Join Jane on this culinary expedition, where nourishing your body becomes a celebration of flavor and well-being. Are you set to embrace the change of
Power of food? Open the cookbook and savor the first chapter of your healthier, more vibrant life.

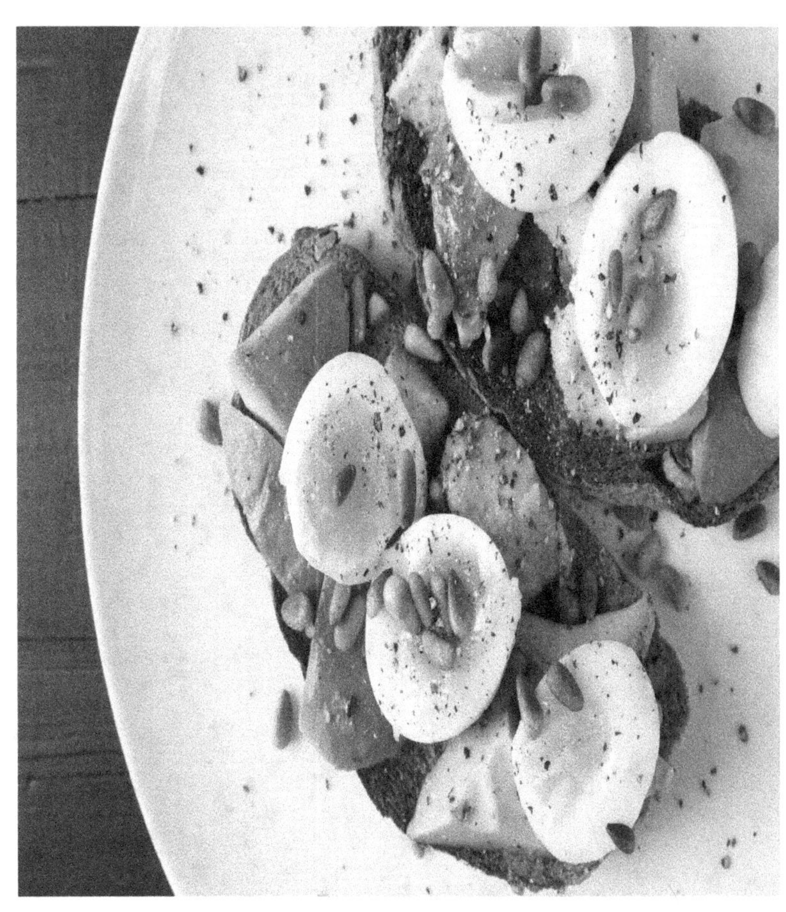

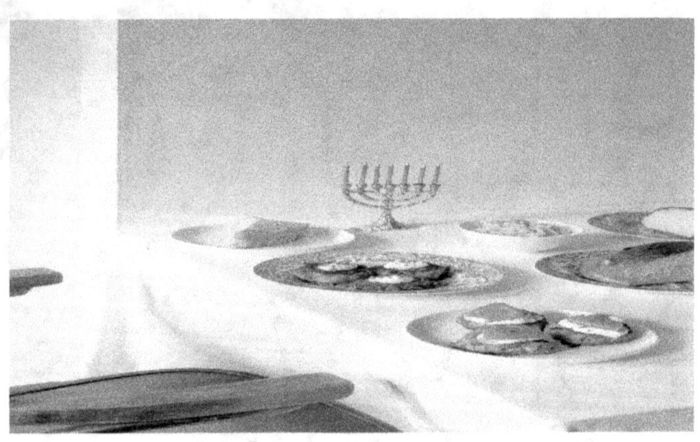

CHAPTER ONE

Exploring the science behind rapid weight loss.

A 10-day diet cookbook explores the scientific concepts underlying swift transformations in the field of rapid weight loss. The fundamental idea is to create a calorie deficit, usually by eating a well-balanced diet and controlling portion sizes. In an effort to increase metabolism and encourage the body to burn stored fat for energy, a high-protein, low-carb diet is recommended. These eating habits frequently make use of thermogenesis, which is the process by which the body produces heat while breaking down food, in order to increase energy expenditure. Nutritionists disagree on whether these quick weight loss techniques are safe and effective. It's critical to acknowledge that these diets may only be temporary and to give priority to long-term, permanent lifestyle adjustments. Prior to starting any fast weight loss program, be sure you know what you want and how desperate you are to go.

Setting realistic expectations

It is essential to comprehend the scientific underpinnings of a 10-day diet when it comes to quick weight loss. These diets frequently adjust caloric intake in order to highlight a caloric deficit. This causes the body to start using its stored energy, which results in weight loss. Additionally, by consuming fewer carbohydrates, these diets may have an impact on water weight. However,Realistic expectations are attainable and doable goals that are founded on a clear knowledge of your capabilities, available resources, and the environment in which you are. It's critical to take into account potential roadblocks and uncertainties in addition to short- and long-term goals.

Setting reasonable expectations will help you feel more accomplished, less stressed, and more satisfied with your work overall. It's critical to evaluate the present state of affairs, acknowledge your limitations, and create a strategy that takes into account both your abilities and the actual conditions.

Many people aim to lose weight quickly—in as little as ten days—but it's critical to understand that balanced approaches are essential in these kinds of attempts. Although the draw of instant gratification may be strong, implementing a balanced approach not only encourages successful weight loss but also places a high priority on general health and wellbeing.

The importance of a balanced approach

A 10-day rapid weight reduction diet that takes a balanced approach has the main advantage of avoiding drastic and unsustainable weight loss methods. Although they frequently have unfavorable side effects, crash diets that emphasize severe calorie restriction or the elimination of entire food groups may result in rapid initial weight loss. Extreme dieting frequently results in exhaustion, muscle loss, and nutrient inadequacies, endangering long-term health as well as short-term success.

A balanced strategy, on the other hand, guarantees that the body gets a wide range of vital nutrients. This consists of a combination of lipids, proteins, carbs, vitamins, and minerals, all of which are essential for maintaining different body processes. For example, proteins help maintain muscle mass, and healthy fats promote satiety and assist the proper functioning of essential organs. Energy is provided by carbohydrates, which promotes weight loss that is sustainable and doesn't jeopardize general health.

A balanced strategy also aids in controlling cravings and maintaining dietary modifications over the ten-day timeframe. People are less likely to feel deprived because they are more likely to find satisfaction in their meals when a variety of foods and flavors are included. This improves adherence to the diet, which is essential for reaching and sustaining weight loss objectives, and makes the plan more pleasurable.An essential component of this strategy is macronutrient balancing. Every nutrient has a specific function in the body, and a well-rounded diet has the right amount of carbohydrates, fats, and proteins. For instance, proteins aid in muscle growth and repair, which is necessary to maintain lean muscle mass when losing weight. Carbohydrates give you energy for daily tasks, while healthy fats help you feel full and absorb nutrients.

Quick fixes frequently result in rebound weight gain once normal eating patterns resume; however, by establishing healthy habits and making gradual, manageable changes, individuals are more likely to maintain their weight loss achievements over time. A balanced approach to a rapid weight loss diet is sustainable in the long run, beyond the immediate benefits.

The importance of a balanced approach in a 10-day rapid weight loss cookbook cannot be overstated. It is a holistic and sustainable way to achieve short-term goals without compromising overall health. By embracing diversity in food choices, balancing macronutrients, and considering the long-term impact of dietary changes, individuals can embark on a rapid weight loss journey that promotes not only a slimmer physique but also a healthier and more resilient body.

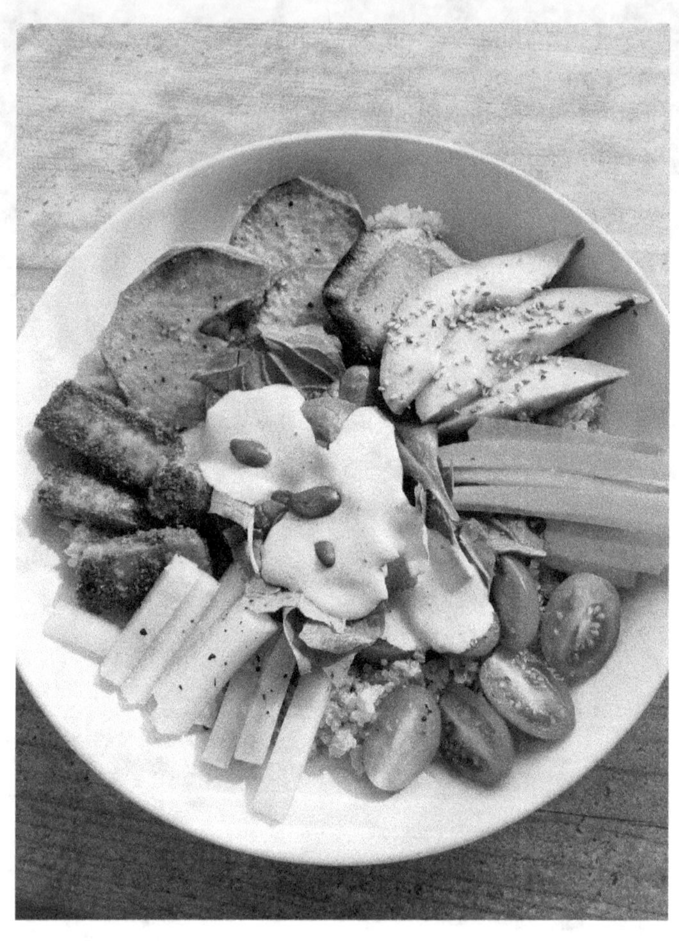

CHAPTER TWO

Assessing your current diet and lifestyle

An essential first step when starting a 10-day rapid weight loss journey with a cookbook is to evaluate your existing food and lifestyle. The first step towards making changes that are long-lasting and successful is understanding your daily routine and eating patterns. To start, record what you eat, when you eat, and how much you eat by maintaining a food journal. This quick look at your current diet tells you what you currently consume in terms of nutrients and where you can make improvements. Make a note of any trends or cues that make you choose bad foods. During your 10-day journey, you can create methods to combat emotional or situational factors by identifying them. Evaluate your degree of physical exercise as well. Frequent exercise promotes general wellbeing in addition to aiding with weight loss. Review your current exercise regimen and think about adding more physical activity to your day.

Once you know exactly what your baseline is, go through the 10-day rapid weight loss cookbook. Seek out dishes that fit your dietary requirements and preferences. Think at how the cookbook approaches nutrition: does it place a strong emphasis on whole foods, portion management, or particular dietary guidelines? Select recipes that fit your objectives and your way of life.

Make a ten-day meal plan that includes a range of nutrient-dense foods. Give fruits and vegetables priority over other macronutrients like proteins, carbs, and fats. The cookbook ought to offer suggestions for meal time and portion levels that will maximize your metabolism and help you lose weight.Keep an eye on your progress during the 10-day adventure. Keep an eye on how your body reacts to the new food and way of living. Keep an eye out for variations in appetite, mood, and energy levels. If necessary, make adjustments to your plan so that it continues to be viable beyond the ten days.

Recall that a 10-day quick weight loss cookbook is only intended to be used temporarily. Use it to spark the development of long-lasting, healthy behaviors. After the ten days, consider the things that went well and the difficulties you encountered. Gaining self-awareness will enable you to make well-informed decisions regarding your nutrition and lifestyle, which will support weight loss as well as general wellbeing.

Creating a personalized plan

A customized 10-day Rapid Weight Loss Cookbook plan must take your nutritional objectives, calorie requirements, and food choices into serious consideration. Here is a little guide to get you going:

1. **Set Achievable Goals:** Establish 10-day weight loss objectives that are doable. Aim for a weight loss pace of 1-2 pounds per week, which is healthy and sustainable.

2. **Find Your Calorie Requirements**
   Based on variables such as age, gender, weight, degree of activity, and weight loss objectives, calculate your daily energy needs. Make sure you have a moderate deficit in calories to lose weight.

3. Select Nutrient-Dense Foods:
   Give special attention to complete, high-nutrient foods including fruits, vegetables, whole grains, lean meats, and healthy fats. These foods encourage fullness while offering vital vitamins and minerals.

4.Preparing Meals:**
   Plan your meals ahead of time to steer clear of bad foods. Make a range of dishes with complex carbohydrates, veggies high in fiber, and lean proteins. Controlling portion size is essential.

5.Hydration:** Make sure you drink lots of water all day long to stay hydrated. Water promotes general wellbeing, decreases hunger, and aids with digestion.

6. Don't Forget Lean Proteins:
   Give priority to lean protein sources such as fish, poultry, tofu, lentils, and turkey. Protein keeps you feeling full and is necessary for the maintenance of muscles.
7. Incorporate Healthful Fats:** Add foods like avocado, almonds, seeds, and olive oil that are good sources of fat. These fats support a balanced diet and offer long-lasting energy.

8. Limit Consuming Processed Foods:
   Reduce your intake of processed and refined foods because they frequently have unhealthy fats and added sugars. Choose entire, unprocessed options if you want greater nutritious content.

9. Time of Meal:**
   For the purpose of sustaining energy levels and managing hunger, think about eating meals in a balanced manner throughout the day. If you need them, include snacks; choose foods high in nutrients.

10. Monitor Progress:** Record the meals, snacks, and general development you've made. If necessary, modify your plan in light of how your body reacts. Remember your objectives and acknowledge little victories.

Setting achievable goals

1. **Set Specific Goals:** Clearly state your 10-day plan for losing weight, taking into account things like your target weight, eating preferences, and any health restrictions.
2. **Portion Control:** To prevent overindulging, emphasize portion sizes. Use visual cues or measurement devices to help you adhere to proper serving sizes.
3. **Incorporate Exercise:** Match an appropriate exercise regimen with your food plan. This combination increases metabolism and improves general health, which facilitates weight loss.
4. Intentional Consumption: Observe the signals your body sends when it is hungry or full. To develop a mindful eating habit, keep yourself from being distracted during meals and enjoy every bite.
5. **Control Stress** : Apply stress-reduction methods such as yoga or meditation. Excessive stress might impede the process of losing weight.

6. **Modify as Required:** Be adaptable and prepared to change your plan in response to your body's reactions. Pay attention to your body and adjust as needed for long-lasting effects.

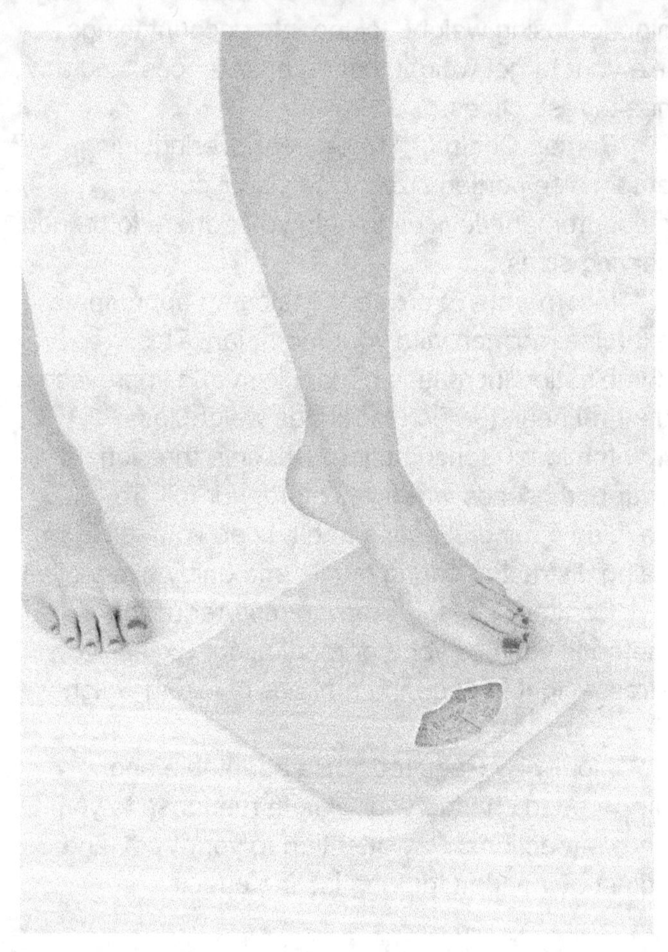

CHAPTER THREE

Daily meal breakdown with calorie counts

Day 1:
- Breakfast:*
 Scrambled eggs with spinach and tomatoes (300 calories)
- Lunch:*
 Grilled chicken salad with mixed greens (400 calories)
- Snack:*
 Apple slices with almond butter (150 calories)
- Evening meal:*
 Baked salmon with asparagus (450 calories)

Compounded: 1300 calories

 Day 2:
- * Breakfast:*
 Poached eggs and avocado on whole grain bread (300 calories)
- *Lunch:*
Brown rice stir-fried with turkey and vegetables (400 calories)
- *Snack:*
 150 calories from a banana and some walnuts
- *Evening meal:*
Zoodle noodles and grilled shrimp (450 calories)

Compounded: 1,300 calories

Day 3:
- * Breakfast:*
 300 calories of oatmeal, fruit, and a teaspoon of
honey
- *Snack:*
An orange and a handful of almonds (150 calories)
-Lunch:
400-calorie grilled chicken breast served with quinoa
and steaming broccoli
* Evening meal:*
 Baked fish served with mixed veggies on the side
(450 calories)

Compounded: 1,300 calories

Day 4:
- Breakfast:
Greek yogurt parfait with granola and mixed berries
(300 calories)
- Snack:
Handful of almonds (150 calories)
- Lunch:
 Quinoa salad with mixed vegetables and grilled
chicken (400 calories)
- Evening meal:
 Baked salmon with asparagus and sweet potato (450
calories)

Compounded: 1,300 calories

Day 5:
- * Breakfast:
Whole-grain bread and scrambled eggs with spinach (300 calories)
- *Snack:
150 calories of mixed berries and Greek yogurt
- *Lunch:
400 calories of grilled chicken salad with mixed vegetables
- *Evening meal:
Baked salmon topped with quinoa and steamed broccoli (450 calories)

Compounded: 1,300 calories

 Day 6:
- * Breakfast:
A 300-calorie Greek yogurt parfait topped with oats and berries
*Snack:
carrot and cucumber sticks with hummus(150 calories)
- *Lunch:
Whole-grain tortilla with turkey and vegetables (400 calories)
- *Evening meal:
 brown rice and stir-fried tofu with a variety of veggies (450 calories)

Compounded: 1,300 calories

Day 7:
Breakfast:*
- Almond milk, chia seeds, and sliced strawberries
added to overnight oats (250 calories)
- One medium peach, or fifty calories (50 calories)

* 400-calorie lunch:*
- Lemon-infused grilled veggie and chickpea
salad-dressing with tahini (300 calories)
- A 100-calorie quinoa and black bean burger

* 150-calorie snack:*
- A tiny handful (150 calories) of walnuts

* Evening meal (450 calories):*
- 300 calories of baked cod with a herb crust
- 150 calories of steamed asparagus spears

Compounded: 1,300 calories

Day 8:

breakfast:*
One small orange (100 calories) and scrambled
eggs with sautéed mushrooms and spinach (200
calories)

* 400-calorie lunch:*
- 300-calorie stir-fried turkey and vegetables with
bell peppers and broccoli.

- One-half cup (100 calories) brown rice

A 150-calorie snack might be cottage cheese and sliced pineapple.

* Evening meal (450 calories):*
- A 300-calorie grilled chicken breast marinated in lemon-herb sauce
- 150 calories worth of roasted sweet potato cubes

Compounded: 1300 calories

Day 9:

* 300-calorie breakfast:*
- One little apple (50 calories) - A smoothie containing kale, banana, protein powder, and almond milk (250 calories)

* 400-calorie lunch:*
- Soup with vegetables and lentils (300 calories)
- A 100-calorie mixed green salad dressed with a light vinaigrette

Snack: 150 calories of Greek yogurt topped with chopped strawberries

* Evening meal (450 calories):*
- A 300-calorie baked fish marinated with lemon and dill.
- 150 calories of steamed broccoli and cauliflower

Compounded: 1,300 calories

Day 10:
* 300-calorie breakfast:*
- One small grapefruit (100 calories) - Whole grain bread with mashed avocado and poached egg (200 calories)

* 400-calorie lunch:*
- A bowl of quinoa and black beans with grilled chicken strips, avocado, and salsa (300 calories)
A 100-calorie side dish of raw baby carrots

Snack: 150 calories of Greek yogurt topped with a few blueberries

* Evening meal (450 calories):*
- 300-calorie grilled shrimp and vegetable stir-fry with bell peppers and broccoli
- 150 calories of steamed asparagus

Compounded: 1300 calories

Well done on finishing the 10-day rapid weight loss plan! When you stop the diet, don't forget to keep eating well and keeping a balanced diet for long-term health.

Nutrient-dense food choices

Look for nutrient-dense foods that are low in calories but abundant in vital vitamins and minerals in a 10-day rapid weight loss plan cookbook. Serve lean proteins, such as fish, poultry, and turkey, with a range of vibrant vegetables and leafy greens. Add legumes, nutritious grains, and nuts and avocados, which are good sources of fat. Reduce your intake of processed foods and added sugars to support a healthy, well-balanced diet for successful weight loss.

Nutrient-dense food choices for a 10-day rapid weight loss diet include:

1. **Lean Proteins:**
   - Chicken breast
   - Turkey
   - Fish (salmon, tuna)
   - Eggs
   - Greek yogurt

2. **Vegetables:**
   - Broccoli
   - Spinach
   - Kale
   - Bell peppers
   - Cauliflower

3. **Fruits:**
   - Berries (blueberries, strawberries)
   - Apples
   - Grapefruit
   - Avocado (yes, it's a fruit!)

4. **Whole Grains:**
   - Quinoa
   - Brown rice
   - Oats
   - Barley
   - Farro

5. **Legumes:**
   - Lentils
   - Chickpeas
   - Black beans

6. **Healthy Fats:**
   - Avocado
   - Nuts (almonds, walnuts)
   - Olive oil

7. **Dairy or Dairy Alternatives:**
   - Greek yogurt
   - Low-fat cheese

8. **Herbs and Spices:**
   - Turmeric
   - Cinnamon

  - Ginger
  - Garlic

9. **Hydration:**
  - Water
  - Herbal teas

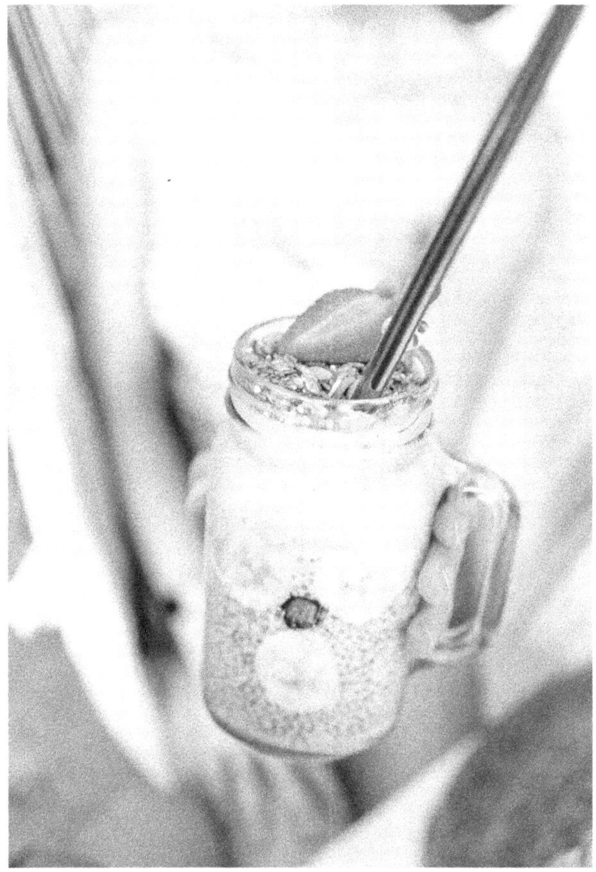

Remember, portion control is essential, and it's crucial to stay within a calorie deficit for weight loss.

Meal Samples

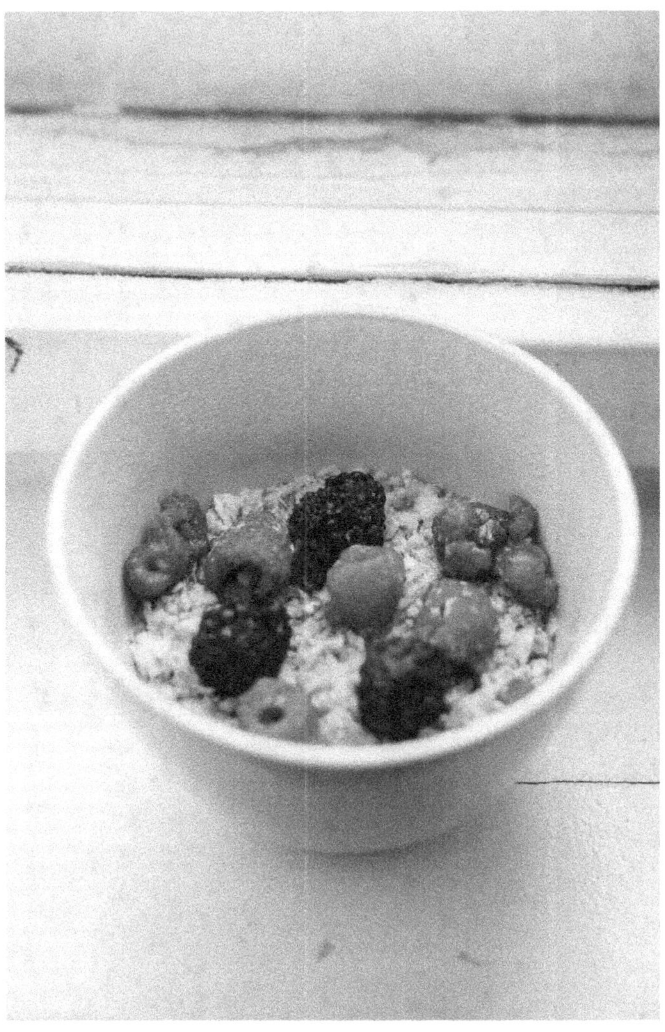

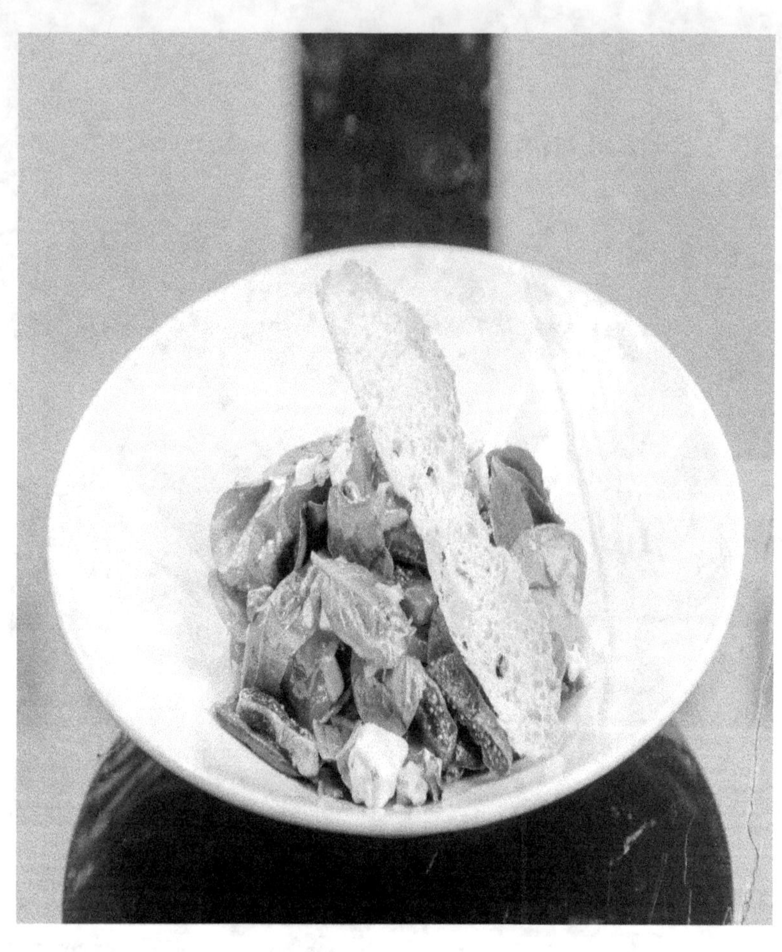

CHAPTER FOUR

Identifying superfoods for accelerated weight loss

1. Leafy Greens:** Spinach, kale, and Swiss chard are rich in nutrients and low in calories.

2. Berries0:** Blueberries, strawberries, and raspberries are packed with antioxidants and fiber.

3. Lean Proteins:** Chicken breast, turkey, tofu, and fish provide protein for muscle preservation.

4. Quinoa:** A protein-rich grain that also contains fiber and essential nutrients.

5. Nuts and Seeds:** Almonds, chia seeds, and flaxseeds offer healthy fats and fiber.

6. Greek Yogurt:** High in protein, it can aid in satiety and support muscle maintenance.

7. Avocado:** Provides healthy fats and can contribute to a feeling of fullness.

8. Green Tea:** Contains antioxidants and may boost metabolism.

Remember, the key to successful weight loss is a combination of a balanced, nutrient-rich diet, regular physical activity, and sustainable lifestyle changes.

Common pitfalls to avoid

1. Extreme Caloric Restriction: Avoid drastically cutting calories, as it can lead to nutrient deficiencies and slow down metabolism.
2. Ignoring Nutrient Balance: Ensure your meals contain a balance of proteins, fats, and carbohydrates to meet nutritional needs.
3. Overlooking Hydration: Stay adequately hydrated; sometimes, thirst is mistaken for hunger.
4. Excessive Reliance on Supplements: Focus on whole foods rather than relying solely on supplements for nutrition.
5. Skipping Meals: Regular meals help maintain metabolism. Missing a meal can cause overindulgence.
6. Lack of Physical Activity: Incorporate exercise for overall health and to enhance weight loss.
7. Short-Term Mindset: View the plan as a jumpstart, not a long-term solution. Sustainable habits are key for lasting results.
8. Ignoring Sleep:Lack of sleep can affect hormones related to hunger and satiety, potentially derailing weight loss efforts.

CHAPTER FIVE

Breakfast delight to consider

Remember, while enjoying these breakfast delights on a 10-day rapid weight loss diet, it's essential to monitor portion sizes and stay mindful of overall calorie intake.

1. Protein-Packed Smoothie Bowl:
   Blend together a mix of low-fat Greek yogurt, a handful of berries, and a scoop of protein powder. Top it with chia seeds, sliced almonds, and a drizzle of honey for a satisfying and nutritious breakfast.

2. Egg White Omelette with Veggies:
   Create a nutrient-rich omelet using egg whites and load it with colorful vegetables like spinach, bell peppers, and tomatoes. Sprinkle with herbs for added flavor without extra calories.

3. Avocado Toast with a Twist:
   Spread mashed avocado on whole-grain toast and sprinkle with red pepper flakes. Top it with

poached eggs for a breakfast that combines
healthy fats, fiber, and protein.

4. Chia Seed Pudding Parfait:
   Combine chia seeds with almond milk and let
them soak overnight. In the morning, layer the chia
pudding with fresh berries and a dollop of low-fat
Greek yogurt for a delicious and filling treat.

5.Turkey and Veggie Breakfast Wrap:
   Wrap lean turkey slices, scrambled egg whites,
and sautéed vegetables in a whole-grain tortilla.
This portable breakfast is rich in protein and fiber.

6. Quinoa Breakfast Bowl:
   Cook quinoa and mix it with almond milk, topped
with sliced bananas, a sprinkle of cinnamon, and a
handful of nuts. Quinoa provides a protein boost
and keeps you full longer.

7. Cottage Cheese and Fruit Bowl:
   Combine low-fat cottage cheese with your
favorite fruits, such as pineapple, berries, and kiwi.
It's a refreshing and protein-packed breakfast
option.

8. Greek Yogurt Parfait:
   Layer non-fat Greek yogurt with granola and
mixed berries for a delightful parfait. This breakfast
is not only tasty but also a great source of protein
and antioxidants.

9. Smoked Salmon Breakfast Bagel:
   Spread light cream cheese on a whole-grain bagel and top it with smoked salmon, capers, and thinly sliced red onions. This savory option provides a good balance of protein and healthy fats.

10. Sweet Potato and Black Bean Hash:
   Sauté diced sweet potatoes, black beans, and veggies like bell peppers and onions. Top it with a poached egg for a nutrient-dense and satisfying breakfast.

Vibrant salads and satisfying soups

For vibrant salads, Here's a sample list of vibrant salads and satisfying soups for a 10-day rapid weight loss diet cookbook:

Vibrant Salads:

1. Kale and Quinoa Power Salad:
   - Ingredients: Kale, quinoa, cherry tomatoes, cucumber, bell peppers, feta cheese, lemon vinaigrette.

2. Spinach and Berry Bliss Salad:
   - Ingredients: Spinach, mixed berries, almonds, goat cheese, balsamic vinaigrette.

3. Mango Avocado Fiesta Salad:
  - Ingredients: Mixed greens, mango chunks, avocado slices, red onion, grilled chicken, cilantro lime dressing.

4. Colorful Mediterranean Salad:
  - Ingredients: Romaine lettuce, cherry tomatoes, olives, red onion, feta cheese, grilled shrimp, Greek dressing.

5. Asian Sesame Ginger Slaw:
  - Ingredients: Napa cabbage, carrots, edamame, red cabbage, sesame seeds, grilled tofu, sesame ginger dressing.

Satisfying Soups:

1. Spicy Lentil and Vegetable Soup:
  - Ingredients: Lentils, carrots, celery, tomatoes, spinach, vegetable broth, cumin, chili flakes.

2. Chicken and Vegetable Quinoa Soup:
  - Ingredients: Chicken breast, quinoa, kale, carrots, celery, low-sodium chicken broth.

3. Tomato Basil Zoodle Soup:
  - Ingredients: Zucchini noodles, tomatoes, garlic, basil, vegetable broth, lean ground turkey.

4. Coconut Curry Chickpea Soup:
   - Ingredients: Chickpeas, coconut milk, curry spices, sweet potatoes, kale, vegetable broth.

5. Mexican Tortilla Soup:
- Ingredients: Black beans, corn, tomatoes, bell peppers, chicken broth, shredded chicken, tortilla strips.

Remember to customize portion sizes based on your dietary needs.

Mouth-watering main courses

1. Grilled Lemon Herb Chicken Breast with Steamed Broccoli
2. Spicy Shrimp and Zucchini Noodles with Garlic Sauce
3. Baked Salmon with Dill and Asparagus Spears
4. Turkey and Vegetable Stir-Fry with Ginger Soy Sauce
5. Quinoa Stuffed Bell Peppers with Lean Ground Turkey
6. Cauliflower Crust Pizza with Tomato, Spinach, and Feta
7. Seared Tuna Steak Salad with Mixed Greens and Citrus Dressing
8. Lean Beef and Vegetable Skewers with Cilantro Lime Marinade

9. Eggplant and Chickpea Curry with Turmeric-infused
Brown Rice
10. Grilled Portobello Mushrooms with Balsamic
Glaze and Roasted Brussels Sprouts.

Guilt-free desserts and snacks

1. Dark Chocolate-Dipped Strawberries
2. Greek Yogurt Parfait with Fresh Berries and
Almond Granola
3. Baked Cinnamon Apple Chips
4. Avocado Chocolate Mousse with a Hint of Vanilla
5. Coconut and Chia Seed Pudding with Mango
Slices
6. Almond Butter Energy Bites with Chia Seeds
7. Mixed Berry Smoothie Bowl with a Sprinkle of
Flaxseed
8. Roasted Cinnamon-Spiced Chickpeas
9. Frozen Banana Bites with a Drizzle of Peanut
Butter
10. Zucchini and Carrot Muffins with a Touch of Honey

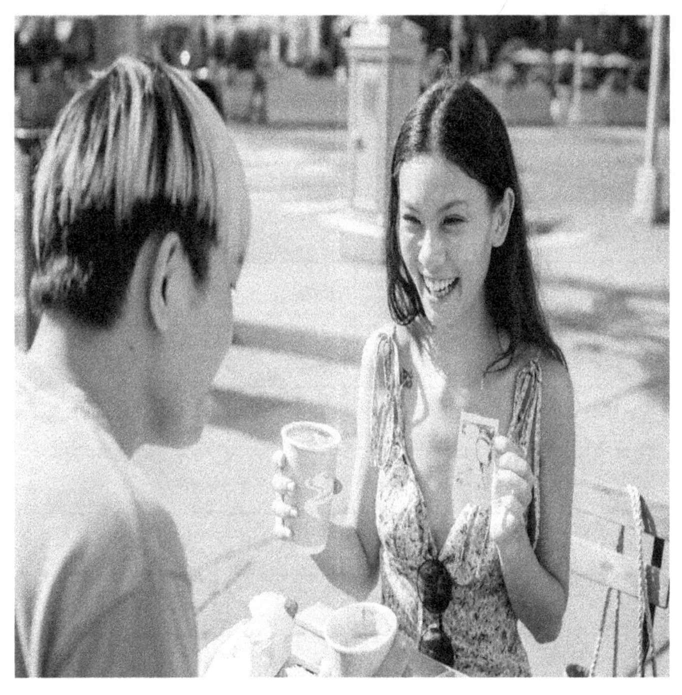

DAY	RECIPES	REMARK

CHAPTER SIX

Complementing your diet with effective workouts

A 10-Day Rapid Weight Loss Diet Cookbook,the synergy of nutritious recipes and dynamic workouts forms a powerful dua for quick and effective results. Each day unfolds a tailored exercise routine, strategically designed to enhance the impact of the accompanying diet plan. From invigorating morning cardio sessions to targeted strength workouts, this cookbook doesn't just guide your meals but propels you through a comprehensive fitness journey. The workouts are crafted to complement the dietary elements, ensuring a harmonious fusion that accelerates fat loss. Whether it's the heart-pumping HIIT sessions or the core-strengthening routines, every exercise is a vital component in sculpting a healthier, leaner you. A 10-Day Rapid Weight Loss Diet Cookbook isn't just a cookbook; it's a holistic approach to rapid weight loss, where the fusion of mindful nutrition and purposeful workouts propels you towards achieving your fitness goals in just 10 days.

Stress management techniques

It is imperative that you incorporate stress management techniques into your 10-day rapid weight loss program. The following techniques will assist you in remaining concentrated and keeping an optimistic outlook:

1. Mindful Eating: Make an effort to be present while you eat. Chew gently, enjoy every bite, and be aware of your body's signals of hunger and fullness. In addition to lowering stress, mindfulness can encourage better eating habits.

2. Take Regular Breaks: Throughout the day, take quick pauses to stretch and unwind. This can ease stress and keep it from building up throughout the peak phase of your fast weight reduction program.

3. Deep Breathing Exercises: To help your nervous system relax, incorporate deep breathing exercises. Try taking four breaths, holding them for four, and then letting out eight breaths. Repeat multiple times to encourage calmness.

4. Drink Plenty of Water: Stress and exhaustion can be exacerbated by dehydration. To maintain your

body and mind operating at their best, make sure you're drinking enough water throughout the day.

5. Quality Sleep: Give adequate, restful sleep top priority. Sleep deprivation might make you more stressed out and hinder your attempts to lose weight. Get seven to nine hours of sleep every night.

6. Physical Activity: To release endorphins, which are organic stress relievers, engage in mild exercise or strolls. This is especially beneficial when going through a phase of high-intensity dieting.

7. Positive Affirmations: Convince yourself of your objectives and acknowledge minor accomplishments. Affirmations that are uplifting can strengthen your resolve and give you more self-assurance.

8. Social Support: Talk to loved ones or friends about your experience so they can offer encouragement. The procedure can be less stressful and more pleasurable if you have a support network.

9. Plan and Prepare: Make sure you have the ingredients you need and plan your meals ahead of time. By being proactive, you can help yourself

maintain your diet and lessen stress at the last minute.

10. Mind-Body Techniques: Take into account implementing techniques like yoga or meditation. These methods can help you become more self-aware and offer a psychological diversion from the difficulties of a quick weight loss plan.

Incorporating these stress-reduction strategies into your 10-day rapid weight loss strategy will improve your general health and raise your chances of meeting your dietary objectives.

Dealing with cravings and emotional eating

Several techniques are needed to control cravings and emotional eating when on a 10-day fast weight loss program. To start, concentrate on including filling, high-nutrient meals from the cookbook. Incorporate a suitable proportion of fiber, protein, and healthy fats to help control blood sugar levels and lessen cravings.

Stay hydrated as well because often thirst is confused with appetite. By focusing on physical hunger indicators rather than emotional triggers, you can practice mindful eating. Find other ways to occupy your time if you feel the need to emotionally eat, such as taking a walk, deep breathing exercises, or taking up a hobby.

Meal planning and preparation can also help you stick to your diet and avoid obsessive eating. Finally, to reduce stress, be realistic about the duration of the diet and set realistic expectations.

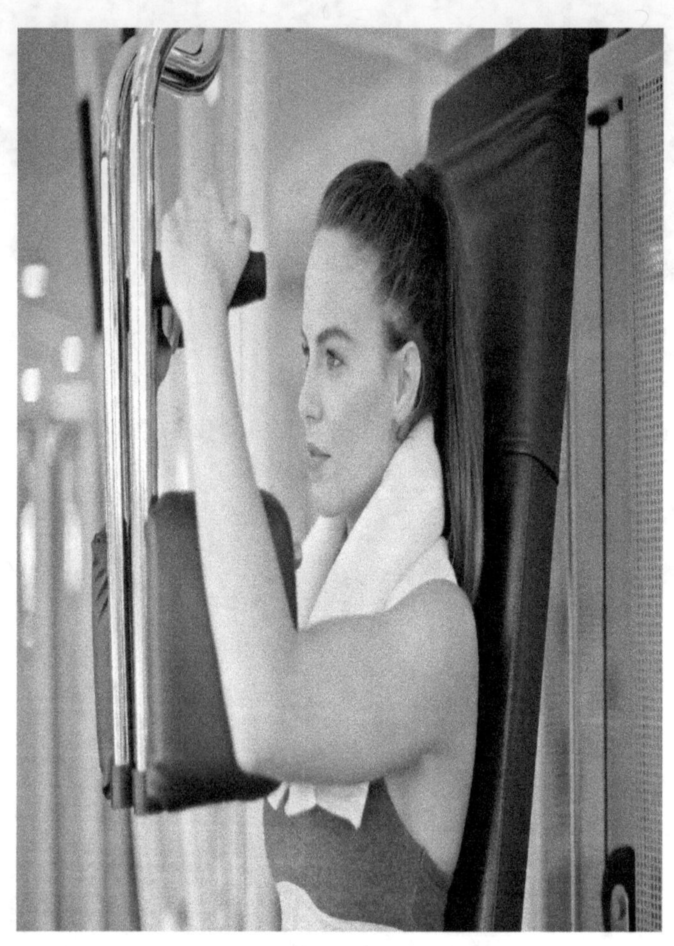

Conclusion

The 10-day rapid weight loss diet cookbook provides a quick solution for shedding pounds, offering diverse and flavorful recipes. However, sustainability is key; relying solely on short-term plans may not ensure lasting results. It's imperative to transition to a well-rounded, nutritious diet for continued health. While these recipes serve as a catalyst, individual needs and long-term habits should be considered.Ultimately, incorporating these recipes into a broader, balanced lifestyle is crucial for achieving and maintaining a healthy weight.